How To Quickly Lose 20 Pounds or More

You Cannot Lose Weight Overnight but

Losing Weight Fast and Easy is Possible

How to Quickly Lose 20 Pounds or More
You Cannot Lose Weight Overnight but Losing Weight Fast and Easy is
Possible
by **Ramon Glyde**

Printed in the United States of America

Legal Notice

Table of Contents

Chapter 1 - Introduction

So you want to take off 20 pounds quick, right? Well, you are not alone. Perhaps you have tried to do this on your own by starving yourself for a week or going on some fad diet. Sure, you'll take off 5 pound right away, but then you find that you reach a plateau and cannot seem to lose the last 5 pounds. Half of the time, you end up gaining a few pounds back and feel more discouraged than ever.

Perhaps you have seen ads for "magic pills" that cost a fortune and promise to melt off your excess pounds without any effort on your part. Save you money. There is only one way to lose weight and keep it off and that is to cut your calorie intake and increase your level of activity. There is no "big secret" to losing weight, but you do have to have the mindset for it. In other words, your desire to lose weight has to be stronger than your desire to eat. With that mindset, you can do anything.

I never had a problem with my weight until I reached 40. At that time I found that I was packing on more weight than ever before. It was also at this time that I quit smoking. I found myself eating more and exercising less. Before I knew it, my clothes were really tight and I had gained an extra 20 pounds, seemingly overnight.

But I wasn't about to go buy new clothes. I had lost weight before. After I had my children I had some extra pounds to lose and took them off right away. So I figured it would be easy to just get rid of 20 extra pounds. So I started a diet and starved myself for a week. I did lose 5 pounds but that was it. I couldn't get the scale to budge after that. And then I came down with a cold.

I wasn't ready to give up. I tried several different methods to lose weight but nothing seemed to work. Then I talked to a friend who I consider to be a weight loss expert. My friend had lost 80 pounds. She confirmed that it takes a while to lose weight, that weight loss does not happen quickly and that it should take four months to lose 20 pounds. But then she let me in on a few secrets of how I can speed up the process and lose 20 pounds in three weeks.

Before you read this book, you should understand that the methods I am recommending to lose 20 pounds in 3 weeks are meant to be for short term weight loss or to jump start a diet. They are not meant to be used on a long term basis. My method of weight loss really does work, I've tried it myself. I lost the weight I wanted to lose and fit comfortably into my clothes again. Last year, when I packed on a few extra pounds over the holidays, I used this method again and it worked again. I have also recommended it to friends who either wanted to get started losing a lot of weight or just wanted to shed some extra weight and it worked for them, too.

Use the methods - all of the methods - that I describe in this book and I guarantee that you are going to lose 20 pounds in 3 weeks.

Chapter 2 - How Weight Loss Works

Before you can lose any weight, you have to understand how weight loss works. Your metabolism a fancy word for your energy level. This is what keeps you going and also burns off calories. Your metabolism continues to work all day long, even when you are sleeping, although it slows down. Think of your metabolism as a motor in your body that has a function of keeping you active and burning off calories.

As you get older, your metabolism slows down. This is why it is much easier to lose weight when you are younger than when you get older. It is the reason why I found it difficult to lose weight in my 40s when I had no problem at all losing baby weight when I was in my 20s. Your metabolism relies on fuel to keep it going. And the earlier in the day you get your metabolism going, the more calories you burn off during the course of the day. This is why we are often told that breakfast is the most important meal of the day.

Some so called "diet experts" say that breakfast

is not important as they try to push pills or fad diets. Not true. While medical science has come a long way in recent years, the basic components of how our bodies work has not changed. The truth of the matter is that you need to boost your metabolism when you want to lose weight. This is why starvation diets do not work. When you starve yourself, your metabolism shuts down. Your body is smart - it knows it is not getting enough fuel so in response, it slows the metabolism to conserve the fuel that it has. You aren't going to lose 20 pounds by starving yourself. But the lack of fuel in your body will lower your immune system and can make you susceptible to colds and other illnesses.

In addition to boosting your metabolism, which I will tell you how to do, you also need to cut your calorie intake. This does not mean that you go hungry, but that you consume the correct amount of calories each day. The purpose of eating is to sustain your body and provide it with the nutrients it needs to function. You never want to consume less than 1200 calories a day or else your metabolism will shut down. You will not feel well, you will be hungry all of the time and just plain uncomfortable. This is not a safe way to lose weight for any length of time, even three weeks. You have to eat, but eating the right foods makes all the difference.

When you cut your calorie intake and increase your metabolism through a variety of different methods, you will lose weight. People who are successful at losing quite a bit of weight understand how this works and follow this method. The only problem with this safe and effective weight loss method is that it tends to work slowly. If you join a weight loss group or seek the guidance of a doctor, you will lose about 1 to 2 pounds a week. This is considered to be a safe way to lose weight.

Trying my method to lose 20 pounds in 3 weeks will enable you to speed up the process. But again, this is meant to be a short term diet. It will work well if you only have 20 pounds that you want to lose, want to jump start a diet or if you have reached a diet plateau when on a weight loss program. It is not meant to be the long term diet for losing a lot of weight.
Now that you understand the simple weight loss process, you are ready to begin to learn how to

lose 20 pounds in 3 weeks.

Chapter 3 - Find Your Ideal Calorie Consumption

The amount of calories that you need to take in each day depends upon your height, your gender, your body type and your activity level. There are hundreds of different calorie consumption guides online that will teach you how many calories you should be consuming each day based upon these factors. There are usually three choices when it comes to activity level - sedentary (which means that you do not exercise much at all), semi-active and very active. You are going to want to use the calories for the sedentary lifestyle, no matter how active you are.

Men tend to lose weight much quicker than women. They also need more calories. Choose your ideal calorie amount that you need to sustain yourself based on these charts. Many of the charts will also tell you how many calories you need to take to lose weight. This will be slightly less than the amount you need to sustain your body. When you find the amount of calories that you need for your body, cut it by

200 calories. For example, let's just say that the calculator tells you that you need to consume 1800 calories a day based upon your height, sex, body type and activity level. You will cut it to 1600 calories a day. This will speed up the weight loss process without making a dramatic change in the amount of food you take in.

Once you understand your calorie limit per day when on this diet to lose 20 pounds in three weeks, you can then figure out calorie consumption. You are consuming calories all of the time, by both drinking and eating. From this moment on, if you expect to lose the 10 pounds in two weeks, every single thing that you put into your mouth has to be accounted for. This includes even tasting food that you are cooking. You do not want to go past the calorie limit that you have set for yourself.

Years ago, you had to buy a book if you wanted to know how many calories were in a piece of chicken or in a hamburger. Today, you can just go on the internet to discover the calories any type of food contains. The more you look them up, the easier it will get for you to understand how many calories you are consuming. Many people who want to lose weight have no idea how many calories are in the foods that they eat and the drinks that they drink. Awareness of calorie intake is one of the key components to losing weight. Once you are aware of what you are eating and how it will impact weight loss, you will be more inclined to choose wisely.

If you stick to the calorie intake per day, when combined with the other aspects of this diet that will be revealed further on in this book, you will be guaranteed to lose 20 pounds in 3 weeks.

Chapter 4 - Foods To Avoid At All Costs

There are literally hundreds of thousands of diet books on the market today. Most of them will give you tips on a certain type of diet. One of the most ridiculous is the Atkins diet. At the same time I was trying to lose 20 pounds, my brother in law was trying to lose about 80 pounds. He went on the Atkins diet before it became well known and insisted that this was the way to go. What happened is that he not only didn't lose the weight, but his cholesterol level shot up. I, on the other hand, lost the weight.

There is no doctor on this Earth who is going to tell you to only eat certain food groups. Fruits and vegetables are good for you and provide nutrients and anti-oxidants that your body needs. While I was eating a sensible diet to lose 20 pounds, my brother in law was consuming Italian sausage without bread and insisting that this was the way to lose weight. That whole concept never made any sense to me then and it still doesn't now. As a matter of fact, sausage is one of the things that you need to avoid when you are trying to lose weight. It is loaded with fat.

The one thing that the Atkins diet did allow me to be aware of, however, was how refined sugars can affect your diet. In the past, if I wanted to take off 5 vanity pounds at the end of winter, I usually skipped taking sugar in my coffee. I was able to lose 5 pounds a week with this just this method alone. I knew sugar added to weight gain as my mother often would talk about candy being "empty calories" in her attempts to lose weight. The Atkins diet brought this to the forefront.

I know what works for me as well as my friends who I recommended this diet to. And that means eliminating all of the following foods from your diet:

Fast foods

A Big Mac has over 500 calories. A medium order of fries has about 400 calories and a coke has 200 calories. Do the math - that is 1100 calories for lunch. Think it's a good idea to super size it?

Fast foods such as fried chicken, pizza and especially fries, should be avoided at all costs when you are trying to lose weight. Most fast foods are not only loaded with fat, but with sodium as well, which allows your body to retail water. They are no good for you. And this includes the Sub sandwiches as well, that are made with processed meats. Pack a lunch from home. If you do eat out, grab a salad. Not a salad that is laced with fried chicken, either. One that is vegetables and perhaps broiled chicken. Use a low fat or no fat dressing.

Above all, skip the fries. These are probably the most devastating to any diet. They offer very little nutritional value, do not really fill you up and are loaded with calories, sodium and fat. For the three weeks that you are on this diet to lose 20 pounds, make a pact with yourself to eat at home or at least bring meals from home. Remember that you are watching your calories and cannot go over your limit. Splurging on fast food may very well put you at the limit for the entire day.

Fried Foods

Everything tastes good when deep fried. In some parts of the world, they deep fry coach roaches and people eat them. And they probably taste good, too. Country singer and actress, Reba McIntyre, has been known to say that "if it ain't fried, it ain't food." While this sounds charming coming from this petite woman, it does not sound good coming from someone who is morbidly obese. Yes, fried food does taste good. It is also filling and cheap. But it just isn't good for you and is loaded with fat and calories. Skip any type of fried food when you are on this diet.

Processed Foods

This includes sausage, lunchmeat and hot dogs, all of which are processed meats. You should also exclude processed cheeses from this diet. Processed foods are simply not good for you - period. They are also high in calories and can ruin your diet. Skip the lunchmeat and replace it with chicken or meat that you make yourself. For example, you can make a meatloaf and slice it very thin for a sandwich instead of having processed meats. It is healthier for you and lower in calories.

Cheese is loaded with fat, but it is also loaded with vitamins that are essential for your health. Real cheese is good for you - processed cheese offers very little by way of nutrition. You want to have a certain amount of dairy in your diet, so real cheese is a better choice than processed cheese. Remember to count your calories.

Frozen Foods

All of those pre-packaged frozen entrees that are made with the diet conscious person in mind should be avoided. They are loaded with sodium. Make your own food - it won't kill you to do this for two weeks. Broil up some chicken breasts and fish on Sunday and make them part of your meals for the week. Boil some hard boiled eggs and use them. Skip the frozen foods as they may promise lower calories, but have a high sodium content.

Condiments

Mayonnaise, ketchup, mustard, salt, barbeque

sauce, salad dressing - all of these have calories that are not taken into account when you are dieting. If you must use condiments in your meals, make sure they are low in fat. Ketchup and mustard are not too bad when used in moderation, but mayonnaise is a killer. It's loaded with fat. If you use any of these condiments, be aware of the calories contained and use them by the teaspoon. Skip the salt entirely.

Sweets

Cakes, cookies, pastries, donuts, candy - all empty calories. No nutritional value and will leave you feeling hungry.   They are a total waste of time and can wreck your diet. If you need to have something sweet to top off your meal, as some people do, then have something like a mint or a small piece of hard candy.   A square of dark chocolate will do as well. Be sure to count this in with your calorie intake.

All of these foods are part of the family of "simple carbohydrates." You have probably heard about the no carbohydrate diets (Atkins is one, the South Beach Diet is another). They are correct in advising people not to eat sweets as they do not stay in your system long enough to offer any nutritional value, are hard on your digestive tract and are quickly absorbed as fat. Where the no carbohydrate diets get it wrong is to lump in all carbohydrates, such as vegetables and fruits, that do have nutritional value.

Fruits can easily be substituted for cake when you want something sweet. Try eating an apple instead of candy after dinner and you will see that this will satisfy your craving for dessert. On top of that, the apple is loaded with nutrients.

By avoiding fast foods, fried foods, processed foods, frozen foods, condiments and sweets, you can expect to lose weight. If, by any chance, you "fall off the wagon" and have a piece of birthday cake, don't beat yourself up. Have just a bite or two of the cake and then go right back on the diet. The secrets that I am sharing with you to allow you to lose 20 pounds in three weeks has a margin of error. Don't beat yourself up if you make a mistake. But at the same time, you have to be aware of your calorie intake and what foods you need to avoid.

Chapter 5 - Watch What You Drink

I have a friend who lost 20 pounds in one month when she stopped drinking cola. Most people today understand that soft drinks are simply liquid candy. They have known this for quite some time, which is why diet sodas were invented. What most people do not realize is that even diet sodas are not good for your diet. The carbonation is difficult for your body to process and the sugar substitutes are not good for your body.

Today there seems to be a trend towards "energy drinks" as well as "health drinks." The former consist of caffeine laden drinks that taste like medicine and the later consist of the latest "super berry" concentrate loaded with sugar. You aren't getting healthy, you are feeding into a money making scheme and paying for fancy bottles of liquid candy. You might as well be drinking a Coke.

I like a cup of coffee in the morning, as do many people. But when you load it up with sugar, cream and coffee syrup, you no longer have a cup of coffee, but a calorie laden dessert. If you want a cup of coffee or a cup of tea in the morning, do yourself a favor and drink it black. If you dislike the taste of the tea or coffee without sugar and cream, then why the heck are you drinking it?

Most people do not realize the amount of calories that they are consuming on a daily basis with their drinks. This includes the morning coffee routine, the drinks you have for lunch and those that you might consume after dinner or when going out for the evening. There are drinks that you need to avoid when you are trying to lose weight and those that you need to have during this process. I'll make it simple for you:

Drinks to avoid

- Alcoholic drinks (these are loaded with sugars)
- Soda of any kind, including diet
- Health drinks like Pomegranate Juice
- Smoothies
- Milk Shakes (this should be obvious)
- Milk

- Fruit juices of any kind

Drinks that you can have

- Water (what a concept)
- Green tea (unsweetened and made by you, not bottled)
- Coffee (one cup a day without cream or sugar - I don't want to torture you)

Let's talk about drinks to avoid first. Okay, you are out on the town and you want to order an alcoholic drink. You have most likely heard that white wine is good for you when on a diet. Wrong! If you absolutely have to have an alcoholic drink, have a dry red wine. This is the alcoholic drink that has the less sugars.

Alcoholic drinks are loaded with sugar and can help you pack on the pounds. We often consider that beer is the alcoholic drink to avoid when we are dieting. Although beer is loaded with sugars and calories, there are some wines that actually top beer when it comes to sugars. Port is one of them.

When you are trying to lose 20 pounds in 3

weeks, avoid alcohol. This is just empty calories that you are taking into your body. If you really can't resist an alcoholic drink for just 3 weeks, you might need a bit more help than just a weight loss program. Do not be fooled into thinking that alcoholic drinks are low in calorie or that they do not matter to your diet. They do.

The same goes for soda. If you truly cannot give up soda for 3 weeks, perhaps you don't want to lose 20 pounds. Although, I'm betting that if you are reading this book that you do. It will not kill you to give up soda for 3 weeks. As a matter of fact, it won't kill you to give it up entirely. Later in this book we will talk about how to keep the 20 pounds off of you by eating and drinking sensibly. Consuming soda on a daily basis is going to add weight.

Fruit juices are mostly made with sugar. I used to think that cranberry juice was really good for you, until I read the label. You are actually better off consuming the fruit or taking a vitamin supplement. Orange juice one of the exceptions. Orange juice that is not made from concentrate is good for you and an excellent source of Vitamin C. You should drink orange juice, but skip it when you are trying to lose 20 pounds in 3 weeks. After that, you can have a juice glass full of this drink each morning to get your metabolism going.

If you do want to take orange juice during this diet, do so in moderation. A small juice glass for breakfast and count it in with your calorie intake. Other fruit juices such as Guava, Pineapple and Apple, as long as they are pure, are also okay in moderation and can be good for you. I am a big advocate of fruits and vegetables and am well aware of their nutritional value. Drinking a juice glass of fruit juice each day is good for you. Drinking glass after glass of sweetened cranberry juice, however, is like drinking soda.

Health drinks are usually loaded with not only sugar, but preservatives as well. They are money makers for those who want to cash in on the latest health craze. If you want a smoothie, make it at home in your blender. Add crushed ice and a fruit, such as blueberries. Blend it up. You are getting the nutrients of the fruit this way and it can be a refreshing drink. Smoothies that are made outside of the home are usually loaded with sugars and fats. If you want a bit more substance in your smoothie, you can add non fat yogurt to the mix. But again, be aware of the calories that you are consuming.

Milk is really good for you and an excellent source of calcium. Unfortunately, it is loaded with fat. Even skim milk is fatty. While you might want to drink milk for bone health, you should skip milk when you are on this diet for 3 weeks. This includes milk shakes, ice cream and other heavy dairy products as well.

Now let's talk about the drinks that you should drink when you are trying to lose 20 pounds in 3 weeks:

Water is like the magic pill for diets. Drinking water is not only good for you, it will boost your metabolism and help you lose weight. We need water to survive. Most people, however, do not drink enough water during the course of the day and get a little dehydrated at times. If you have ever felt thirsty, this is a sign of dehydration.

If you drink 6 to 8 glasses of water each day,

you will boost your metabolism and aid in weight loss. Once you get used to drinking water, you will also find that it tends to keep you healthier as it flushes toxins out of your system. Do you want to lose 20 pounds in 3 weeks? Then substitute water for your every day drinks.

Coffee and tea is something that many of us like in the morning. You should limit your coffee and tea consumption to one cup per day as too much caffeine gives you a false high and ends up sending you crashing. Also, coffee is very acidity and difficult on the stomach. If you cannot stomach coffee or tea without sugar or cream, you should switch to….water! Water will actually give you the same energy boost that you get from coffee.

Green tea has been in the news recently and has been embraced by diet gurus as a "miracle" drink. It is not a miracle drink and does contain caffeine. But it is not the same type of caffeine found in black tea or coffee. You can drink green tea, unsweetened, either cold or hot. You should brew it yourself at home as when you purchase bottles of this drink in the store, it is usually loaded with sweeteners and artificial preservatives that totally negate any health advantages of the drink.

If you find water to be too bland to drink though out the day, you might want to add some green tea to your diet. Green tea that you brew yourself and drink without sugar either hot or cold does not have any calories. You can drink this drink and it will boost up your metabolism in the same way that water will do so.

Personally, I like green tea and have not had any problems sleeping when drinking this drink. If you are not used to caffeine, however, you might try this in small doses. The caffeine boost that you get from green tea is supposed to raise your metabolism so that you burn more calories. But I have tried this diet with both water and green tea and have not found any difference when it comes to weight loss. So while green tea is not the "miracle" diet aid that some people claim it to be, it is beneficial when you are trying to lose weight.

Drink 6 to 8 glasses of water or unsweetened green tea each day and you will be able to lose 20 pounds in 3 weeks if you use these drinks to replace other drinks that you are consuming.

Another trick for dieting that you can use is to drink a glass of water before each meal. This has the means to fill you up before the meal and cause you to eat less. Do not underestimate the power of water to help you lose weight.

Chapter 6 - Boost Your Metabolism

I have talked about foods and drinks through much of this book but very little about metabolism. While it is essential to eat right when you are trying to lose weight, it is also imperative that you boost your metabolism. Your metabolism will burn calories and allow you to lose fat.

So how do you give your metabolism the boost that it needs? One way is by eating foods that are high in proteins, eating them early in the day and drinking plenty of water. All three will boost your metabolism. Then, of course, there is the "E" word. This is the one word that people who are trying to lose weight never want to hear. It is also very misunderstood. The word, of course, is exercise. This is what many diet gurus and those pushing "magic" pills will tell you that you can avoid when trying to lose weight.

Trying to lose weight, any amount of weight, without exercise is a colossal waste of time. The good news about exercise is that it happens to be the "magic" potion that you need not only to lose weight, but also to maintain good physical and mental health.

Each year after the New Year, millions of people nationwide make a pilgrimage to health clubs everywhere, signing up for lifetime memberships with the intent to "get healthy" after binging incessantly during the holiday season. By March, most people have given up on the health club and are not going regularly. Attendance at the health club continues to dwindle and eventually drop off completely. Until January when the entire process starts again.

Each year, millions of people purchase expensive exercise equipment for their homes and pay large monthly installments to keep this equipment. This also occurs around January. And by March, many people have very expensive clothes hangers or dust collectors in their house. You can usually find many of these items at garage sales by the summer.

The point I am trying to make is that exercise is not something that you should do on a whim to try to lose weight - it should be a part of your life. And you don't need to have expensive equipment or join a gym to exercise. Any increase in physical activity on a daily basis will enable you to not only lose weight, but also to feel better. You will find that exercise not only increases your metabolism, but it also gives your immune system a boost.

You do not have to buy equipment or join a club to exercise. And you can use exercise to both boost your metabolism as well as relax you before bed. You can do this right in the privacy of your own home, or close to home, simply by understanding the importance of activity as well as how cardiovascular exercise and stretching can work.

The reason that many people fail at exercising, which is actually a very simple concept, is that they tend to overdo it when they start out. In an effort to lose as much weight as possible, they end up over exerting themselves on machines or at the health club and pull muscles. They also fail to warm up properly or cool down properly as well. This tends to defeat the purpose of exercise as you will be forced to be sedentary while your muscles heal.

You have probably heard that you should not exercise close to bedtime or right after a meal. This is true when it comes to cardiovascular exercises, which are designed to get your circulatory system pumping and allow you to burn fat. You do not want to do this before bed as it will give you a burst of energy that may make it difficult for you to fall asleep.

Exercise can give you a natural source of energy that is better than any so called "energy drink" on the market. And it has no calories or chemicals. It is one thing that is easy to do and is good for you in a variety of different ways. Even if you have a difficult time getting around, you can still participate in some form of cardiovascular exercise.

One form of cardiovascular exercise that will help you lose weight, give you a burst of energy and also alleviate stress (which is a big factor in why many people are overweight) is brisk walking. Taking a brisk walk around the block in the morning before you go to work will get your metabolism working right away and help you burn fat throughout the day. If you are not a morning person and find it difficult to get up a half an hour earlier in the morning to do this quick walk around your block, you can do this when you get home from work. A brisk walk is one of the best ways to perform cardiovascular exercising and is low impact.

Low impact means that it is easy on your knees and back. As we get older, our joints start to stiffen up, making exercising more difficult. Think back when you were a kid and had tons of energy. You never walked anywhere, you ran. You played all day outside, running around, and still had energy to spare. This is not so with adults. As we age, our metabolism slows down, we find we have less energy and it gets more difficult to exercise. When we do not use our muscles for long periods of time except to flip the remote switch on the TV, they tend to get stiff. This makes exercising more difficult.

If you want to lose 20 pounds in 3 weeks, you have to increase your level of physical activity. The easiest way to do this is to take a brisk walk in the morning. Getting your motor running early is the best way to lose weight and is essential for quick weight loss. If you are like most people, however, your morning routine goes something like this:

Alarm goes off, you hit the snooze button and sleep as long as possible.
You put the coffee on and hit the shower to get ready for work.
You get dressed, groomed and drink a cup of coffee while getting ready to leave.
You do not allow any time for anything else, you are on a tight schedule. You get ready and maybe take a cup of coffee with you when you are heading out the door.
You rush to work either bucking traffic or taking a train. You might stop for more coffee.
You get to work and then settle at your desk. Your body feels like it is just starting to wake up as you get yet another cup of coffee.

Does that sound like you? You're far from alone. This is how most people start their day. Then they wonder why they are stressed out and tired all the time. If you tell someone that they should exercise in the morning, the first thing they will say is that they "don't have time."

Think about it - you have time to take a shower and get fixed up for work, right? You have time to put a pot of coffee on, right? Exercise in the morning should be just as important to your health and well being as taking a morning shower and should take precedence over the coffee. Try this routine instead:

Alarm goes off 10 minutes ahead of schedule. You actually get up and toss on some sweats. Dressed for the weather, you head out your door and take a brisk walk around your block for 10 minutes.
You shower and groom, getting ready for work. You drink a glass of water and eat instant oatmeal for breakfast without the sugar (you can sweeten it with pure maple syrup or honey which is less fattening).
You head out the door and drive to work, feeling a lot more energetic. Okay, you can take your coffee with you.
You get to work and feel more awake, less grumpy and ready to work. You drink another glass of water while you are at work.

The first scenario will not aid you in losing

weight. The second scenario can make all the difference and can easily help you lose 20 pounds in 3 weeks. Oatmeal is a good whole grain that is also good for your heart. You are giving your body fuel and boosting your metabolism with food, exercise and water. You can take two people and give them the same diet and activity for the rest of the day, and the one who starts the day off with scenario two will lose more weight and be in better shape than the person who practices scenario one. Not only will they be in better shape physically, but mentally as well.

Exercise gets your motor going. Feeding the motor with fuel (the oatmeal, for example) does not take a long time and will actually help you burn more calories throughout the day. Remember that your metabolism is always burning calories, even when you are traveling to work. When it is revved up, it burns them faster. This is why a good morning routine is essential if you want to lose weight.

Now if you are just not a morning person, you can still help yourself by exercising when you get home from work. You should still eat something in the morning that is good for you (a boiled egg is another excellent way to start the day) to boost your metabolism. Your body has shut down for the night and your metabolism has slowed down. In order to rev it up, you need to give it fuel. That is why breakfast is given its name. You are breaking the fast. You are giving your body the energy it needs to start your engines and burn off calories.

Any type of exercise that gets your heart pumping such as running, jogging, speed walking, walking, stair climbing, can be considered cardiovascular exercise. You do not have to overdo it. You do have to increase the level if you are going to lose weight. If you have been used to jogging in the morning, for example, you should either jog for a longer period of time or run. The main thing that you want to remember when you exercise is that you want to increase your level of activity to enable your body to burn more calories.

Walking is the best exercise for someone who is used to being inactive. It is low impact and will still manage to boost your metabolism. You can walk at a brisk pace and get your motor going.

If you can do this in the morning, the weight loss will be easier.

Get into a routine when it comes to exercise and make it easy on yourself. Start out slowly and gradually build up your routine. As the pounds start to come off and you feel better about how you look, you will start to look forward to your routine and will also be able to increase your level of activity. Not only will you be able to lose weight, but you will feel more energized throughout the day.

If you are planning on running or doing strenuous exercise, make sure that you warm up first by doing a series of stretching exercises. This will get your muscles ready for exercise and decrease the chances of causing damage to the muscles. You can lose 20 pounds in 3 weeks without overdoing it when it comes to exercise.

Exercise can also be used as a way to relax you so that you get a good night's sleep. Many people today are so stressed that they complain of trouble sleeping. Take a few minutes each night to do some stretching and some yoga exercises and you will feel more relaxed before bed time and will get a better night of sleep.

While we are on the subject of sleeping, it is also a good idea to try to maintain a regular sleeping schedule when you are trying to lose weight. This is actually a good idea for anyone. You should try to go to bed around the same time each night and wake up the same time each morning. This is good for your internal body clock and will aid in regulating your metabolism.

So, while it is important exercise when you are trying to lose 20 pounds in 3 weeks, you do not have to buy a gym membership, get fancy equipment or over exert yourself. You just have to increase your level of physical activity through some form of cardiovascular exercise, preferably in the morning, in order to lose weight.

After you have lost the 20 pounds that you want to lose, do not give up on exercise. You should continue to take your walks and perform relaxing stretching techniques as this is a good way for you to not only keep the weight off, but also stay physically and mentally healthy as well.

Chapter 7 - Mind Over Matter

This book has basically taught you that in order to lose 20 pounds in 3 weeks, you have to cut your calorie intake and increase your physical activity. Common sense, right? You can get this advice from others and probably already have. Later in this book, I will give you a day by day routine that you can follow to get the weight off as promised. But there is more to losing weight than just following directions. Something that most diet books never discuss.

Losing weight is easier than you think. It is simply mind over matter. Your desire to lose weight has to be greater than your desire to eat. Many people who are overweight go on diets to lose the weight, but do not ever grasp the bigger picture, which is why you are overweight.

If you are seeking to lose 20 pounds in three weeks, chances are that you are looking for a way to look better in your clothes which might be a bit too tight due to indulging during the holidays, a time when most of us go on what can only be described as an eating frenzy.

Gaining an additional 20 pounds during this time is no big deal, but it is good to take off the weight so that you can stay in your clothes.

But many people who are overweight are where they are due to a number of different factors. Food becomes a source of solace for them. It stops being a means to survive and becomes the reason for survival. Food is fuel. It is necessary for our survival. Sure, we all like to eat a good meal and enjoy snacks, but when food becomes a central focus in your life, it is time to re-evaluate your life and why you are giving food more prominence in your life than it deserves.

I had an acquaintance at a former job who was obese and was desperate to lose weight. She tried a number of different diets and kept falling off the diet wagon. Every day she would lament over two things - the fact that she was overweight and the fact that she was single. She looked at her weight as an obstacle to her happiness. Looking back on this, she never talked about anything else.

Even when she was on a diet, she was

consumed with food. I can remember her coming into the office one day with chocolate chip bread she had made the night before. She was so proud of herself for not indulging in the food and gave it to the rest of the staff in the office. I can remember thinking that she was very masochistic for doing this. After all, there was no occasion for her to make this bread. She was just obsessed with food.

She was overweight, but very attractive. She was also intelligent and a nice person. Yet she did not go out on dates with guys who asked her as she was waiting for her weight loss to transform her into a more desirable person. She had no hobbies or interests besides food and losing weight.

One of the things that people who are trying to lose weight need to understand is that nothing magical happens when you lose weight. You are still the same person. One of the biggest secrets to losing weight is to get your mind off of food and start getting consumed with living your life. Do not wait for weight loss to allow your life to begin, start living it now. You will find that the more attention you start paying to other things, such as hobbies, friends, etc., the less attention you will focus on your weight and eating.

If you get a chance, rent the movie "Fatso" starring Dom Deluise. This charming movie illustrates my point perfectly about mind over matter. The central character, played by Deluise, is an obese bachelor who lives to eat. Concerned after the death of a cousin of a sudden heart attack, who was also overweight and the same age as him, he goes to a diet doctor and embarks on a diet. This makes him want food all the more. The movie focuses on him struggling to lose weight and losing the battle as he cannot overcome his food addiction. He meets a woman who likes him for who he is and starts enjoying his life with her, resigned to the fact that he is fat, but happy.

But a funny thing happens. He finds that he is losing weight without even knowing it. He stops focusing on food and starts focusing on life as he wants it to be and winds up losing weight. I wish my former work acquaintance would have taken a cue from this movie.

The bottom line is that if you want to lose 20 pounds in 3 weeks, practice the diet and exercise tips in this book, but do not become consumed with food or weight loss. Do not wait until you have lost weight to begin living your life, start doing it right away. You will find that the less you focus on food and the more you focus on other aspects of your life, the easier it is to lose weight.

Chapter 8 - Falling Off The Diet Wagon

Chances are that after reading this book, you will be all geared up to lose weight. You will have the formula for doing so and be ready to take off 20 pounds in 3 weeks. So what happens when, after a few days, you get tempted with a piece of cake or some other treat? What happens if you wake up late one morning and do not have time to take your walk? In other words, what do you do when you fall off the wagon?

One of the reasons why many people fail at dieting is because they fall off the wagon. This is a term that is used often to describe alcoholics who start drinking after being sober for a period of time, but it can be used when describing any type of addiction and a break from the routine of trying to overcome bad habits. Many people get very discouraged when they fall off the wagon, to the point that they decide that the entire idea has to be scrapped. Fear of failing again can keep them from even trying to continue with the diet or the healthy lifestyle choice that they have made for themselves. So they go back into their familiar routine, despite the fact that it was not working for them.

If you fall off the wagon while you are practicing this diet, forget it. You made a mistake and ate a piece of cake or didn't exercise for a day - so what? Everyone makes mistakes. This does not mean that you are a failure. Just get right back into the groove and continue with the plan as if nothing happens. Beating yourself up over a mistake that you made does nothing to help you. Once piece of cake will not sabotage your diet. But giving up because you had that piece of cake will destroy all that you worked for.

Do not be afraid of failure. Continue to persist with your healthy lifestyle choice, despite setbacks. Do not view a deviation as a colossal failure, but a slight setback in what you want to do and continue on with your goal. If you have to add another day onto the diet plan because you splurged at a party, so what? Just get back on the wagon as soon as possible and continue down the path that you have chosen for yourself.

Chapter 9 - Average Diet Ideas

So, now you are ready to start your diet and lose 20 pounds in three weeks. You already know what foods that you have to avoid as well as what not to drink. You should have some sort of exercise routine planned for yourself so that you increase you level of activity. Here are some tips on what you can eat throughout the day to keep yourself nourished:

Breakfast

Remember that breakfast is the most important meal of the day. This is actually where you want to consume the most calorie. Breakfast ideas for a diet include cereal that is unsweetened such as Special K and Cheerios. Measure the cereal into a bowl and watch your calorie intake. Use skim milk for your cereal and, if possible, add fresh fruit. Blueberries are not only low in calories when compared to other fruits, but they are also very nutritious and high in antioxidants.

Eggs are often criticized for being high in

cholesterol, but they are an excellent source of protein. You can have an egg for breakfast as long as you cook it properly. Soft boiled eggs are good as are hard boiled eggs. You will not want to eat fried eggs or use butter in any way.

If you like toast, you can eat a slice of whole grain wheat toast with fruit preserves. Use a teaspoon to measure the preserves so that you do indulge too much. You can also spread the toast with low fat peanut butter. Again, use a teaspoon and measure the calories. You will want to keep your calorie intake to about 300 calories for breakfast.

Oatmeal is very good and can be sweetened with honey, which is low in fat, or even maple syrup. Pure maple syrup should be used and not corn syrup, which is high in calories. Oatmeal is very good for maintaining good cholesterol, if filling and works well to get your morning started off on the right foot.

Skip the breakfast bars. They are high in calories, preservatives and fat. If you truly do not want to take time to make breakfast and eat it at home, then take a banana with you on your way to work. A nutrition bar has about 250 calories, a banana has about 70.

You will find, after you have eaten a breakfast, that you will be hungrier for lunch than you would be if you skip breakfast altogether. This is good - it means your metabolism has kicked in and that you are burning calories. Your body is looking for fuel.

Snack

Have a mid morning snack. You can have a number of different things, but they should be measured and the calories counted. An apple is a good source of vitamins, takes a few minutes to eat and can be filling. Be sure to drink plenty of water throughout the morning to continue to keep your metabolism going.

Raisins are also a very good healthy snack, but be mindful of the sugar content. Many so called healthy snack packs like trail mixes are actually very high in calories. Sunflower seeds, unsalted, are a good source of protein. A mid morning snack will take the edge off of your hunger and help you so that you do not overindulge in your lunch.

Lunch

Salads are good for lunch. By this time, you have probably consumed about 400 calories. Your lunch should be something that you brought from home or a salad at a local restaurant.   Use a vinegar salad dressing instead of ranch as it is lower in calories. If you can, try eating a salad with just vinegar. I did this once for a week and lost 5 pounds without doing anything else. Vinegar has hardly any calories at all.   Salad dressing, on the other hand, can totally wreck your diet.

Oranges are a good source of nutrition and can be good for after lunch. The sweet flavor of the orange will top off the meal and give you a feeling of satisfaction and because they take a while to peel, this will also keep you from being tempted into eating more. Again, you will want to continue drinking water throughout the day, especially with your meals.

Low fat cottage cheese or, better yet, Ricotta cheese, is an excellent source of protein and can be eaten for lunch. The same with low fat yogurt. You have a variety of choices when it comes to you lunch and you can have up to 400 calories. At the end of lunch, you should not still feel hungry.

Snack

Although people scoff at "rabbit food" diets, raw celery and carrots are not only good for you, but they have hardly any calories at all. You do not even have to worry about the calorie intake of celery raw as you burn more calories chewing it than it contains.

When you are snacking after lunch, be sure to stay away from salty snacks such as crackers, as they can cause you to retain water. You will notice the weight starting to come off in the first two days of the diet, although much of this will be water weight. You will also notice that you will be making more trips to the bathroom. This is good as you are flushing the fat (and toxins) out of your system.

Dinner

You want to keep your calories down during dinner and it should be your last meal of the day. You will find that the more you eat in the morning, the less you will feel you need to eat for dinner. You can have a normal dinner with the family, just watch the portions. Keep your calorie intake to the limit and skip dessert. Be mindful of how the meal is cooked. Substitute olive oil for other fats and broil instead of other fats.

One way that you can enjoy dinner without feeling as though you are depriving the entire family as well as yourself is to simply cut your portions in half. Drink a glass of water before the meal to make yourself feel the need to eat less. Eat slowly and chew your food more instead of wolfing it down. This will take you longer to eat and will allow you to feel content in a shorter period of time.

You should, after each meal or snack, feel satisfied and not full. Many people feel that in order to be satisfied with a meal, they have to feel full. You do not want to feel full, you simply do not want to feel hungry. The secret to successful dieting, especially when you are seeking to lose a lot of weight in a short amount of time, is to eat until you are no longer hungry but not until you are full.

By understanding how many calories you are consuming as compared to how many you need, you have a leg up on losing weight. The more you are aware of the calories in the foods that you are eating and the foods that you need to avoid, the easier dieting will become.

I did not want to write a book that gives you details on exactly how much to eat and what on which day as this rarely works. Not everyone has the same tastes when it comes to food and not everyone needs the same amount of calories. The trick is to eat foods that are good for you and will provide you with the nutrition that you need to maintain your body. If the foods that I have listed do not appeal to you, then eat the foods that you normally eat and simply cut the portions in half. Eat breakfast, drink plenty of water and exercise. You will lose the weight if you follow this outline.

To make it even simpler, here is the blueprint of what you have to do to lose 20 pounds in 3 weeks:

- Find out how many calories you need to sustain yourself based on your body type, height, activity level and gender;
- Use the sedentary scale for calories you need and cut it by 200;
- **Eat breakfast!**
- Increase your exercise level by performing cardiovascular exercises such as speed walking for at least 10 minutes each day;
- Eliminate fast foods, fried foods, processed foods, sweets, and frozen foods from your diet;
- Drink water or unsweetened green tea instead of any other drink and avoid alcohol;
- Drink 6-8 glasses of water or green tea each day;
- Consume steady calories throughout the day instead of all in one meal.

This is pretty much all you need to do if you want to lose 20 pounds in 3 weeks. Stick with this routine for three weeks and you will have dropped at least 20 pounds. Some people who have used this diet routine have lost up to 15 pounds in two weeks.

Remember that this is meant to be a short term diet. If you want to continue to lose weight after you have lost the 20 pounds, you should look to a long term diet and do not expect to lose 7 pounds a week. It is safe, when dieting on a long term basis, to lose 2 pounds a week.

Stick with the diet and remember that your desire to lose 20 pounds has to exceed your desire to eat. Think of how proud you will be of yourself when you have achieved your weight loss. It is a good idea, to keep yourself motivated in losing weight, to give yourself some sort of reward when you have accomplished your goal.

Remember that if you get sidetracked and end up falling off the wagon, to just pick yourself up and get right back on track. Do not beat yourself up over a mishap - it is in the past and there is nothing that you can do to move time backwards. Concentrate on the future and moving forward.

Chapter 10 - Keeping The Weight Off

If you follow the tips that I have outlined in this book, you will lose 20 pounds in 3 weeks, guaranteed. You will feel good about this accomplishment as well and you might even lose a size or two in your clothing. The trick is now to keep the weight off.

One thing that you should do is to continue with the exercise routine. This is crucial to keeping the weight off that you have lost. Change is very difficult for most people, even when it is positive change. You might find yourself slipping back into your former routine and eating foods that are not good for you. If you find that you are doing this, stop and get right back on the right path.

You may love fried foods and long for chicken and French fries. You can have them, and ice cream, too. Just remember that they are very high in calorie content and fat and cut your normal portion of these items. Remember to eat until you are no longer hungry and not until you are stuffed to the point that you can no longer move.

Do not obsess over weight gain of a pound or so. You might want to increase your activity so that you can take off that pound, but we all tend to fluctuate with our weight by a few pounds. Hopefully, after you have read this book and succeeded in taking off the 20 pounds, you will have a better understanding of how to eat, what to eat and what not to eat. This can make losing additional weight much easier than you may have imagined.

Continuing to eat a healthy diet, avoiding foods that are not nutritious and provide you with nothing but empty calories and exercising is the way to keep those 20 pounds off. Not only will you look better and your clothes fit you much nicer, but you will also feel better both mentally and physically. Once you continue with the healthy eating habits as outlined in this book, you will find that you do not have to concentrate so hard on watching your weight as you will be able to naturally maintain it.

Remember to keep your eyes on the prize. Your mind is your best motivational diet tool, so do not underestimate its power. Focus on other aspects of your life other than food and maintain your desire to stay at your ideal weight, making it more important than your desire for food. Congratulations on your weight loss and good luck in keeping it off in the future!

www.ingramcontent.com/pod-product-compliance
Lightning Source LLC
Chambersburg PA
CBHW081418280526
45788CB00009B/3148